The Rules For Obesity Understanding the Science Behind Weight and Wellness

By

Christa Winter

Table Of contents

Introduction

Key points
*Adiposity, which refers to
abnormal or excessive body fat,
is a common, complex,

progressive, and recurrent chronic condition that harms health.

*Independent of weight or body mass index, the stigma and discrimination experienced by those who live with obesity contribute to higher rates of morbidity and mortality.

*This updated set of guidelines takes into account significant developments in epidemiology, pathophysiology, assessment, prevention, and treatment of obesity. It also changes the emphasis of obesity management away from weight loss alone and toward improving patient-centered health outcomes.

*Obesity care should be founded on evidence-based methods of managing chronic diseases, validate patients' lived experiences, go beyond the basic advice to "eat less, move more," and address the underlying causes of obesity.

Access to evidence-based interventions, such as medical nutrition therapy, physical exercise, psychiatric interventions, medication, and surgery, should be available to people who are obese.

Adiposity, an abnormal or excessive amount of body fat, affects health, raises the possibility of long-term medical consequences, and shortens lifespan in obesity, a complicated chronic condition.1 Body mass index (BMI; weight/height2), which may classify obesity-related health risks at the population level, is the measure of obesity used in epidemiologic investigations. BMI of more than 30 kg/m2 is the operational definition of obesity, and it is further divided into three classes: class 1 (30-34.9), class 2 (35-39.9), and class 3 (40). At the population level, the health risks associated with high body fat rise as BMI does.2 At the individual level, difficulties arise as a result of excessive fat accumulation, the location and distribution of fat, and a variety of other factors, such as socioeconomic, genetic, biological, and environmental ones (Box 1).11

Box 1:
Obesity-related complications
In addition to having an impact on the body's ability to regulate its internal energy balance, adipose tissue can become dysfunctional and increase a person's risk of developing a wide range of health issues, including:
* Type 2 diabetes3
*Gallstone illness 4
*Non-alcoholic fatty liver illness 5
*Gout6
Excess and ectopic body fat are significant sources of

adipocytokines, which are inflammatory mediators that can change how glucose and fats are metabolized. This can raise the risk of cancer and cardiometabolic disease and shorten life expectancy by 6 to 14 years.1,7,8 Independent of nutrition, it is believed that obesity causes 20% of all malignancies.9 The risk of the following malignancies is increased by obesity:
*Colon (both sexes)
*Kidney (all sexes)
* Esophagus (Both sexes)
*Endometrium (women)
*Postmenopausal Breast (Women)
The frequency of obesity has continuously climbed over the past three decades all across the world,12 and it has tripled in Canada since 1985.13 Importantly, the number of Canadian adults who suffer from extreme obesity has more than quadrupled and affected 1.9 million people in 2016.13 Obesity has emerged as a significant public health problem that drives up medical expenses (14, 15) and has detrimental

effects on one's physical and mental well-being.16 Obesity-related stigma and bias are prevalent, and they raise morbidity and mortality rates (regardless of weight or BMI).17 The complex interaction of numerous genetic, metabolic, behavioral, and environmental factors that contribute to obesity is what causes it. Environmental factors are assumed to be the direct cause of the significant increase in the prevalence of obesity.18,19 In recent years, it has become clearer what the biological causes of this disease are.19 By controlling food intake and energy usage, the brain is a key player in maintaining energy balance (Box 2).24

Box 2:
Controlling appetite 20–23

*A complex brain network, including the hypothalamus (homeostatic regulation), the mesolimbic system (hedonic control), and the frontal cortex (executive control), work together to regulate appetite.

*Adipose tissue, the pancreas, the gut, and other organs all produce mediators that have an impact on the interaction between homeostatic and hedonic eating.

*Executive control over dietary decisions and the decision to eat is exerted by cognitive processes in the prefrontal cortex. These brain networks' connectivity, which regulates eating behavior, has been found to change in obese people.

A negative energy balance is caused by a reduction in food intake and an increase in physical activity, which sets off a series of metabolic and neurohormonal adaptation mechanisms.[25,26] The long-term management of obesity may benefit from treatments that focus on these changes in neurohormonal systems.[27]

In clinical practice, new methods for diagnosing and rating obesity have been put forth.[11,18,19,28] Although BMI is frequently used to evaluate and categorize obesity (adiposity), it is not a reliable measure for finding issues associated with adiposity.[19] Independent research has linked an increase in waist circumference cardiovascular risk instead.29 When BMI and waist circumference are combined, it may be possible to detect the higher-risk phenotype of obesity more accurately than either metric alone, especially in people with lower BMIs.30,31 A thorough history to determine the underlying reasons for obesity, an adequate physical examination, and pertinent laboratory tests may help to identify people who will benefit from therapy in addition to BMI and waist circumference measurements.32

The Edmonton obesity staging system has been proposed (Appendix 1, available at www.cmaj.ca/lookup/suppl/doi:1 0.1503/cmaj.191707/-/DC2).28 The best way to manage obesity is determined by this five-stage classification method for obesity, which takes into account metabolic, physical, and psychological factors. It has been demonstrated in population studies that, when compared to BMI or waist circumference measurements alone, it is a more

accurate predictor of all-cause mortality.33,34
There is an understanding that managing obesity should focus on bettering health and well-being rather than just weight loss.34-36 Many of the suggestions in this guideline are weight-loss focused because the majority of the existing literature is based on weight-loss results. However, additional research is required to reorient obesity management away from weight loss alone and toward enhancing patient-centered health outcomes. Despite mounting evidence that obesity is a major chronic disease, our existing healthcare system is ineffective at managing it. Health workers in Canada report feeling underprepared to assist obese patients.39-41 Biased attitudes toward fat also impact the quantity and caliber of medical care that obese patients receive.42 Because of the prevalent societal narrative surrounding obesity, persons who are obese are blamed for their condition and are treated with contempt.41 Importantly, the level and quality of care

provided to persons who are obese are significantly impacted by the stigma around obesity.42 The 2006 Canadian clinical practice guideline should be updated given the advancements in our understanding of the disease state and better methods for assessing and managing obesity.43 The purpose of this update is to provide primary care physicians with evidence-based choices for diagnosing and managing obese patients. This recommendation makes important use of the viewpoints of interprofessional primary care practitioners, persons with lived experience, experts in the management of obesity, and researchers. The whole policy is available online, and this article provides a synopsis of it.

Scope

The main healthcare providers are the intended users of this recommendation. In addition to those impacted by obesity and their families, policymakers may also use the recommendation.

The focus of the recommendation is adult obesity. All those who follow the suggestions should exercise clinical judgment; they are meant to be a guide for healthcare professionals. Although it may be challenging to implement every piece of advice due to resource constraints and patient choices, the goal of the guideline is to raise the caliber and accessibility of care for people with obesity across Canada.
Recommendations
The primary care setting's clinical management strategy and patient journey are both informed by this clinical practice guideline. Table 1 displays the suggestions for the guidelines.

Table 1:Recommendations for treating adult obesity

The strength of the suggestion and the category of evidence lowering the prevalence of weight bias in obesity management, practice, and policy 1 Health professionals should evaluate their attitudes and beliefs about obesity and think about how such attitudes and beliefs might affect the way they give care. Grade A, level 1a

2 Healthcare professionals may be aware that internalized weight bias, or bias against oneself, among obese people, can have an impact on behavior and health outcomes. B level, level 2a

3 When working with patients who are obese, healthcare professionals should refrain from utilizing judgmental language (level 1a, grade A), visuals (level 2b, grade B), and behaviors (level 2a, grade B). Refer to advice

4 We advise healthcare professionals to refrain from assuming a patient's illness or complaint is connected to their body weight. Gradel C, level 3.

Obesity epidemiology in adults

5 Healthcare professionals can identify and treat obesity as a chronic disease that is brought on by an abnormal or excessive buildup of body fat (adiposity), which compromises health and increases the risk of premature morbidity and mortality. Grade B, level 2b.

6 Adult obesity can be managed through the development of evidence-based solutions at the health system and policy levels. Grade B, level 2b.

7 Regularly collected self-reported and measurable data (such as height, weight, and waist circumference) may be used in continued longitudinal national and regional surveillance of obesity. Grade B, level 2b.

enabling those who live with obesity to participate in daily activities

8 We advise health care professionals to inquire about patients' concerns on managing self-care activities such as washing, dressing, managing bowel and bladder function, caring for their skin and wounds, and caring for their feet. Grade C, level 3.

9 Because obesity may limit a person's capacity for and interest in physical activity, it is advised that healthcare professionals evaluate a patient's fall risk. Grade C, level 3.

evaluation of those who are obese

10 We recommend that healthcare professionals who are involved in the screening, assessment, and management of patients with obesity use the 5As framework (see Appendix 2) to start the conversation by obtaining their consent and determining whether they are ready to start treatment. Level 4, consensus grade D

11 Medical professionals can measure a person's height, weight, and BMI in all adults (level 2a, grade B), as well as their waist circumference in those with a BMI of 25 to 35 kg/m2 (level 2b, grade B). Refer to advice

We advise that the assessment include a thorough history to pinpoint the underlying causes of weight gain, as well as any problems from obesity and potential therapy roadblocks. At level 4, a D

13 To assess cardiometabolic risk in obese individuals, we advise taking measurements of blood pressure in both arms, fasting glucose or glycated hemoglobin, lipid profile, and, when necessary, ALT to screen

for nonalcoholic fatty liver disease. tier three, grade D

14 To assess the degree of obesity and direct clinical decision-making, healthcare professionals may think about adopting the Edmonton Obesity Staging System (see Appendix 1).At level 4, a D

The importance of mental health in managing obesity

We advise routine weight, glucose, and lipid profile monitoring in patients with a mental health diagnosis who are also using weight-gaining medicines. Grade C, level 3.

16 When selecting psychiatric drugs, healthcare providers may take into account both efficacy and effects on body weight. B level, level 2a

17 People with severe mental illness who are being treated with antipsychotic drugs related to weight gain should take into consideration metformin and psychological therapies such as cognitive behavioral therapy to minimize weight gain. Grade A, level 1a

18 Medical professionals should think about using

lisdexamfetamine and topiramate
as a supplement to psychological
treatment to help persons with
binge eating disorders and
overweight or obesity lose
weight and reduce eating
pathologies. Grade A, level 1a
Medical nutrition therapy for the
treatment of obesity
19 To support a dietary approach
that is safe, effective,
nutritionally adequate, culturally
acceptable, and inexpensive for
long-term adherence, we propose
that nutrition guidelines for
adults of all body sizes be
tailored to fit individual values,
preferences, and treatment goals.
At level 4, a D
20 Individualized medical
nutrition therapy administered by
a licensed dietitian (where
available) should be given to
adults who are obese to enhance
weight outcomes (body weight,
BMI), waist circumference,
glycemic management, set
cholesterol, and blood pressure
targets.Grade A, level 1a
When a registered dietitian is
available, adults with obesity,
impaired glucose tolerance
(prediabetes), or type 2 diabetes

may undergo medical nutrition therapy to lower body weight, reduce waist circumference, and improve glycemic control and blood pressure. B level, level 2a
22 Adults with obesity can choose the dietary regimens and food-based strategies that will promote their best long-term adherence when considering any of the several medical nutrition interventions to enhance health-related outcomes. (Full recommendation, type of evidence, and level of evidence are accessible in the chapter headed "Medical nutrition therapy in obesity management.")
23 To improve glycemic control, blood pressure and blood lipid targets (level 1a, grade A), and to reduce the incidence of type 2 diabetes (level 1a, grade A), microvascular complications (retinopathy, nephropathy, and neuropathy) (level 1a, grade B), cardiovascular and all-cause mortality (level 1a, grade B), adults with obesity and impaired glucose tolerance should think about intensive behavioral

interventions that target a 5%-7% weight loss. Refer to advice
24 To raise the remission of type 2 diabetes and lower the incidence of nephropathy, obstructive sleep apnea, and depression, adults with obesity and type 2 diabetes should think about rigorous lifestyle therapies that aim for a 7%–15% weight loss.Grade A, level 1a
25 To improve cardiovascular results, quality of life, psychological outcomes (general well-being, body image perceptions), body weight, physical activity, cognitive restraint, and eating behaviors, we advise against dieting. Grade C, level 3.

Management of obesity with exercise

26 Adults who want to Lose weight can think about aerobic physical exercise (30-60 minutes of moderate to intense intensity most days of the week).
*Lose fat and body weight in tiny amounts (level 2a, grade B)

even in the absence of weight loss, reduce ectopic fat, such as liver and heart fat, and visceral fat in the abdomen (level 1a, grade A).
*Favor maintaining weight after losing weight (level 2a, grade B)
*Favor maintaining lean body mass when losing weight (level 2a, grade B)
*Improve mobility (level 2a, grade B)
* cardiorespiratory fitness (level 2a, grade B).

Refer to advice

27 Resistance training may help individuals who are overweight or obese maintain their weight or modestly increase their muscle mass, fat-free mass, or mobility. B level, level 2a

28 Increasing the intensity of an exercise program, such as high-intensity interval training, can result in higher increases in cardiorespiratory fitness and shorter times
to reap the same benefits as moderate-intensity aerobic exercise. B level, level 2a

29 Many cardiometabolic risk variables in people with overweight or obesity can be

improved by regular physical exercise, with or without weight loss, including hyperglycemia and insulin sensitivity (level 2b, grade B), high blood pressure (level 1a, grade B), and dyslipidemia (level 2a, grade B). Refer to advice
30 Adults who are overweight or obese can benefit from regular physical activity in terms of health-related quality of life, mood disorders (such as depression and anxiety), and body image. Grade B, level 2b.

Effective behavioral and psychological therapies for the control of obesity

31 Care plans for weight loss, improved health status, and quality of life (level 1a, grade A) should include multicomponent psychological interventions that combine behavior modification (goal-setting, self-monitoring, problem-solving), cognitive therapy (reframing), and values-based strategies to alter diet and activity in a way that encourages

adherence, confidence, and intrinsic motivation (level 1b, grade A).

Refer to advice

To support the development of self-efficacy and intrinsic motivation (personal, meaningful reasons to change), healthcare providers should provide people with obesity longitudinal care with consistent messaging. They should also encourage patients to set and sequence health goals that are realistic and achievable, to self-monitor their behavior, and to analyze setbacks using problem-solving and adaptive thinking (cognitive reframing).Grade A, level 1a

33 Healthcare professionals should seek the consent of those who are obese before explaining to them that managing obesity successfully depends more on achieving behavioral goals that will enhance one's health, function, and quality of life than it does on how much weight is lost. Grade A, level 1a

To foster the growth of self-efficacy and intrinsic motivation. 34 Healthcare practitioners should conduct follow-up sessions that are consistent with repetition and relevance. Level 1a, grade A (Full recommendation may be found in the chapter headed "Effective psychological and behavioral interventions in obesity management").

Pharmacotherapy for the treatment of obesity

Liraglutide 3.0 mg, naltrexone-bupropion combination, orlistat are some examples of medications that can be used in conjunction with medical nutrition therapy, physical exercise, and psychological interventions to help people lose weight. B level, level 2a

36 Liraglutide 3.0 mg or orlistat may be used as a pharmacotherapy to sustain weight reduction that has been attained by healthy behavior modifications and to prevent weight return. B level, level 2a

37 Liraglutide 3.0 mg (level 1a, grade A), naltrexone-bupropion combination (level 2a, grade B), and orlistat (level 2a, grade B) are three examples of medications that can be used in conjunction with behavioral

changes in health for people with type 2 diabetes whose BMI is less than 27 kg/m2. Refer to advice

38 Liraglutide 3.0 mg; orlistat is recommended for use in conjunction with health behavior changes for patients with prediabetes, overweight, or obesity (BMI 27 kg/m2). This can help to postpone or avoid the onset of type 2 diabetes. B level, level 2a

39 Other than those that have been approved for weight control, we do not recommend using prescription or over-the-counter drugs. Level 4, consensus grade D

40 For persons who are overweight or obese and need pharmacotherapy for other health issues, we advise selecting medications that are not linked to weight gain. Level 4, consensus grade D

Preoperative evaluation and selection for bariatric surgery

41 We advise patients for bariatric surgery to have a thorough medical and nutritional screening and any nutrient

deficits should be treated. At level 4, a D

42 Quitting smoking before surgery helps reduce perioperative and postoperative problems. B level, level 2a

43 For those considering having bariatric surgery, we advise testing for and treating obstructive sleep apnea. At level 4, a D

Bariatric surgery: operative possibilities and results

44 People with a BMI of less than 40 kg/m2 or a BMI of less than 35 kg/m2 who have at least one adiposity-related condition (level 4, grade D, consensus) may want to consider having bariatric surgery to:

Lower the overall long-term mortality rate (level 2b, grade B).

better long-term weight loss than medical management alone (level 1a, grade A)

Increase the effectiveness of best medical management in bringing type 2 diabetes under control and into remission compared to best medical management alone (level 2a, grade B)

increase life quality significantly (level 3, grade C)

Most adiposity-related illnesses, such as dyslipidemia (level 3, grade C), hypertension (level 3, grade C), liver steatosis, and nonalcoholic steatohepatitis (level 3, grade C), can be brought into long-term remission.

Refer to advice

45 Patients with poorly managed type 2 diabetes and class I obesity (BMI between 30 and 35 kg/m2) should be evaluated for bariatric surgery.Grade A, level 1a

46 People with class 1 obesity who have tried everything, even the best medical and behavioral therapy, have failed to significantly reduce their weight. Bariatric surgery may be an option. B level, level 2a

47 We advise collaborating with an experienced interprofessional team to choose the best bariatric treatment (sleeve gastrectomy, gastric bypass, or duodenal switch) based on the patient's needs. Level 4, consensus grade D

48 Due to undesirable consequences and long-term failure, we advise against

offering adjustable gastric bands. At level 4, a D

49 Due to long-term problems compared to Roux-en-Y gastric bypass, we advise against frequently providing single anastomosis gastric bypass. At level 4, a D

Surgery for weight loss: postoperative care

Providers of healthcare can encourage bariatric surgery patients to take part in and make the most of their access to behavioral treatments and allied health services at a bariatric surgical center. B level, level 2a

51 We recommend that, for patients who are discharged, bariatric surgical centers communicate a thorough care plan to primary care providers that details the procedure, emergency contacts, required yearly blood tests, long-term vitamin and mineral supplements, medications, and behavioral interventions, as well as when to refer back. Level 4, consensus grade D

52 After a patient has left the bariatric surgical center, we advise primary care doctors to

review their weight, nutritional intake, activity level, compliance with multivitamin and mineral supplements, evaluation of comorbidities, and laboratory tests to identify and address nutritional deficiencies as needed. Level 4, consensus grade D

53 For technical or gastrointestinal symptoms, nutritional concerns, pregnancy, psychological support, weight regain, or other medical issues related to bariatric surgery, as described in the chapter titled "Bariatric surgery: postoperative management," we advise primary care providers to consider referring back to the bariatric surgical center or a local specialist. Level 4, consensus grade D

54 It is recommended by us that bariatric surgical centers offer postoperative follow-up and appropriate laboratory tests at regular intervals, along with access to the proper health care professionals (dietitian, nurse, social worker, bariatric physician, surgeon, psychologist, or psychiatrist), up until the

patient's discharge is deemed appropriate. Level 4, consensus grade D

Primary health care and primary care in the treatment of obesity

55 We advise primary care physicians to recognize patients who are overweight or obese and to start patient-centered, health-focused interactions with them. Grade C, level 3.

56 We advise medical professionals to make sure they obtain consent from patients before discussing weight or performing anthropometric measures. Grade C, level 3.

57 As an efficient intervention to manage weight, primary care treatments should be used to improve health literacy in people's knowledge and abilities about weight management. Grade A, level 1a

58 To support the management of obesity, primary care practitioners should refer people who are overweight or obese to multi-component primary care programs with individualized obesity management techniques.Grade B, level 1b.

59 To support improved physical and emotional health as well as weight management, primary care doctors can employ collaborative deliberation in conjunction with motivational interviewing to design action plans for each individual's living context in a way that is manageable and sustainable.Level 2b, C-level

60 Interventions that are directed towards a particular ethnic group should take into account the variety of psychological and social norms relating to obesity, eating habits, and physical activity, as well as socioeconomic conditions, as these may vary across and within different ethnic groups. Grade B, level 1b.

61 To effectively support people in managing their weight, longitudinal primary care interventions should concentrate on gradual, individualized, minor behavioral improvements (the "small change approach"). Grade B, level 1b.

Personalized obesity management solutions are an efficient way for primary care

multi-component programs to
serve patients who are obese.
Grade B, level 1b.
To control overweight and
obesity, primary care
interventions that are behavior-
based (nutrition, exercise,
lifestyle), either alone or in
combination with medicine,
should be used. Grade A, level
1a
Adults with overweight and
obesity should employ group-
based diet and exercise sessions
that are informed by the Diabetes
Prevention Program and the
Look AHEAD (Action for
Health in Diabetes) programs as
an efficient management option.
A level, level 1b
65 In a community-based
environment, interventions that
make use of technology to
enhance access to larger numbers
of people asynchronously should
be a potentially viable lower-cost
intervention. Grade B, level 1b.
66 Courses and clinical
experiences for primary health
care professionals should address
the gaps in skills, knowledge of
the evidence, and attitudes
necessary to confidently and

effectively support people living with obesity. These courses should be offered in undergraduate, graduate, and continuing education programs. Grade A, level 1a

Commercial weight-loss goods and initiatives

67 When compared to standard care or education, the following commercial programs should help adults who are overweight or obese lose mild to moderate amounts of weight in the short or medium term:

Weight Watchers (previously WW) (level 1a, grade A)

*(Level 1b, Grade B) Optifast

*Jenny Craig (grade B, level 1b)

*Nutrisystem (grade B, level 1b)

Refer to advice

68 When compared to standard counseling, Optifast, Jenny Craig, WW (formerly Weight Watchers), and Nutrisystem should mildly lower glycated hemoglobin values over a short period in adults with obesity and type 2 diabetes. Grade B, level 1b.

69 Due to a lack of data, we do not advise using over-the-counter commercial weight-loss products

to manage obesity. At level 4, a
D.

70 We do not advocate using
commercial weight-loss
programs to help adults with
obesity control their blood
pressure or lipid levels. At level
4, a D

**Virtual medicine and emerging
technologies in the treatment of
obesity**

71 For the management of
obesity, management strategies
can be implemented via web-
based platforms (such as online
education on medical nutrition
therapy and physical activity) or
mobile devices (such as daily
weight reporting via a
smartphone application). B level,
level 2a

72 To improve the results of
weight loss, we advise medical
professionals to incorporate
personalized feedback and
follow-up into technology-based
management strategies (such as
personalized coaching or
feedback via phone or email).At
level 4, a D

73 A comprehensive weight
management plan should include
the use of wearable activity-

tracking technology. Grade A, level 1a

Weight control during the reproductive years for adult obese women

We advise primary care physicians to talk to adult women with obesity about weight-management goals specific to the reproductive years: preconception weight loss (level 3, grade C); gestational weight gain of 5 to 9 kg throughout the entire pregnancy (level 4, grade D); and postpartum weight loss of — at least — gestational weight gain (level 3, grade C) to lower the risk of negative outcomes in the current or future pregnancy. **Refer to advice** 74 For adult women with obesity who are considering becoming pregnant (level 3, grade C), who are pregnant (level 2a, grade B), and who are postpartum (level 1a, grade A).

75 primary care providers should provide behavior change interventions that include both nutrition and physical activity. Refer to advice

76 To help pregnant women with obesity achieve their desired

gestational weight gain, primary care providers should encourage and support them to eat foods that fit into a healthy dietary pattern. Grade C, level 3.

77 To help with the management of gestational weight gain, primary care providers should encourage and support pregnant obese women who do not have medical conditions that prevent them from exercising while pregnant to engage in at least 150 minutes per week of moderate-intensity physical activity. Grade C, level 3.

78 Pregnant patients with obesity (level 1b, grade A) should not be given metformin for gestational weight gain. We advise against using weight-management drugs while nursing or while pregnant (level 4, grade D). **Refer to advice**

79 Due to lower rates of initiation and continuation, we advise providing additional breastfeeding support to women who are obese. Grade C, level 3.

Obesity Management and Indigenous Peoples

80 We suggest that healthcare providers for Indigenous people living with obesity:

*Engage with the patient's social realities.

*Validate the patient's experiences of stress and systemic disadvantage influencing poor health and obesity, exploring elements of their environment where reduced stress could shift behaviors.

*Advocate for access to obesity-management resources within publicly financed healthcare systems, acknowledging that resources beyond may be pricey and inaccessible for many.

*Help patients know that excellent health is achievable and that they are entitled to it.

*Negotiate small, realistic milestones pertinent to the patient's context.

*Address resistance, seeming apathy, and paralysis in patients and providers.

*Self-reflect on anti-Indigenous sentiment frequent within health care systems, analyzing patient motives and mental health (e.g., trauma, sorrow) as alternative understandings of reasons and remedies to their health problems. Explore one's capacity for bias impacted by institutional racism.

*Expect patient mistrust in health systems; reposition themselves as a helper to the patient instead of as an expert, which may generate opposition and be a barrier to patients' wellness.

*When resistance, seeming apathy, and paralysis are encountered, evaluate the patient's mental and emotional health issues, which have specific drives and presentations in many Indigenous cultures.

*Build complex knowledge via healing connections.

*Build patient knowledge and ability for obesity self-management through longitudinal studies of co-occurring health, social, environmental, and cultural determinants. Strive to develop connections that encompass healing from multigenerational trauma that, owing to residential schools and child welfare system participation, may more frequently entail sexual assault.

*Build their knowledge of the health legacy of colonization — including current experiences of anti-Indigenous discrimination within systems and wider society — to facilitate connections built on mutual understanding.
*Ensure the knowledge offered is aligned with the patient's viewpoints and educational level, and is learner-centered, including the potential for patient anticipation of racism or uneven treatment.
*Connect to conduct, the body, and Indigenous ways of knowing, doing, and being.
*Elicit and include the patient's individual and community-based notions of health and healthy behaviors about body size, exercise, and food preferences (e.g., preference for or scarce access to land-based foods and activities).
*Engage deeply in the study of shared ideals and rules for dialogue and information-sharing in indigenous cultures (such as relationalism and non-interference).

ALT stands for alanine aminotransferase, and BMI is for body mass index.

*A detailed explanation of the guidelines and the supporting data can be found at http://obesitycanada.ca/guidelines/. The actionable verbs used in these recommendations are defined in Table 3.

†See Box 3 for the classification system for evidence category and strength.

‡Visit www.cmaj.ca/lookup/suppl/doi:10.1503/cmaj.191707/-/DC2 to access Appendix 2. Look at Appendix 1.

The 19 chapters of the comprehensive guideline (obesitycanada.ca/guidelines/) provide a detailed explanation of the suggestions and supporting data. The executive committee's discussion of the guiding concepts it believes are crucial for enhancing clinical practice in Canada is summarized in this overview.

The patient arc consists of five steps that might help a healthcare professional treat obese patients. Following are summaries of the

pertinent suggestions and
discussions of supporting data
for each step.
1 Recognition of obesity as a
chronic illness by medical
professionals, who should
request the patient's consent
before providing advice or aiding
in the objective treatment of this
illness,
2 evaluating a person who is
obese, taking accurate measures,
and figuring out the underlying
causes, problems, and treatment
hurdles.
3 Discussion of the primary
forms of therapy (medical dietary
therapy and physical exercise) as
well as any possible
supplemental treatments, such as
psychological, pharmaceutical,
and surgical measures
4 Agreement on the therapeutic
objectives with the obese person,
with an emphasis on the benefits
that person gets from health-
based therapies.
5 The involvement of health care
professionals in ongoing follow-
up and reassessments with obese
patients as well as
encouragement of advocacy to

enhance care for this chronic illness

Step 1 : Recognizing obesity as a chronic illness and getting the patient's consent are the first steps.

Primary care physicians should recognize and treat obesity as a chronic condition with an increased risk of premature morbidity and mortality that is brought on by abnormal or excessive body fat accumulation (adiposity).1,2,18,44-47

Like any other complex chronic disease, obesity is a complex and heterogeneous condition that requires specialized care and ongoing support. Obesity does not manifest itself in all patients in the same way.

The quality of care provided to patients who are obese can be compromised by weight bias in health care settings.42 Being conscious of one's attitudes and behaviors toward people who are obese is important for minimizing weight bias, stigma, and discrimination among healthcare professionals.48 This can be accomplished by completing a self-assessment instrument for weight bias, such as the Implicit Association Test.49 The chapter titled "Reducing Weight Bias in obesity management, practice, and policy" can be found online (obesitycanada.ca/guidelines/) and provides a thorough explanation and supporting data for the weight bias suggestions. Healthcare professionals shouldn't presume that all obese individuals are ready to start managing their obesity. Once the patient has given their consent to talk about their obesity, the health care professional can start talking about possible treatments.50,51

Step 2: Evaluation

To prevent stigmatizing and too-simplified narratives, primary care physicians should encourage a holistic approach to health with an emphasis on health behaviors in all patients and cautiously address the core reasons for weight gain.

All individuals should undergo a routine medical checkup that includes exact measurements of their height, weight, and waist circumference, as well as the

BMI calculation. Although BMI has its limits, it is nonetheless a useful measure for population health indices and screening purposes.52 Waist circumference should be periodically assessed in people with elevated BMIs (between 25 mg/m2 and 34.9 mg/m2) to identify people with elevated visceral adiposity and adiposity-related health concerns.53

In addition to sociocultural practices and beliefs, social determinants of health, the built environment, personal life experiences like adverse childhood experiences, and psychological factors like mood, anxiety, binge-eating disorder, attention-deficit/hyperactivity disorder, self-worth, and identity, the root causes of obesity also include biological factors like genetics, epigenetics, neurohormonal mechanisms, associated chronic diseases, and obesogenic medications.50 Personalized plans can be created by working with people to comprehend their context and culture, as well as to incorporate their core reasons. These strategies can be incorporated into long-term treatment partnerships with chronic illness follow-up for obesity and associated comorbidities, including addressing the underlying factors that contribute to obesity, such as pre existing diseases and obesogenic drugs. We advise acquiring a thorough history to find these fundamental reasons for weight increase as well as any physical, psychological, or psychosocial obstacles. Based on clinical judgment, a physical examination, laboratory tests, diagnostic imaging, and other investigations should be conducted. To assess cardiometabolic risk, we also advise testing blood pressure in both arms, obtaining fasting glucose or glycated hemoglobin levels, a lipid panel, and, if necessary, an alanine aminotransferase test to check for nonalcoholic fatty liver disease.

Step 3: A discussion of available therapies

Individualized treatment plans should be provided to adults who are obese and address the underlying reasons for their condition. These plans should also support behavioral changes (such as improving nutrition and physical exercise) and complementary therapy, which may include psychological, pharmaceutical, and surgical interventions.

exercising and eating Everyone would benefit from adopting a healthy, well-balanced eating pattern and partaking in regular physical activity, regardless of their body size or composition. A minor amount of weight and fat reduction, improvement in cardiometabolic parameters, and weight maintenance following weight loss can all be attributed to aerobic exercise (30–60 minutes) most days of the week.54

Long-term calorie restriction is necessary for both weight loss and weight maintenance. Managing health and weight requires long-term adherence to a healthy eating pattern that is tailored to each individual's beliefs and tastes while also meeting nutritional needs and treatment objectives.

The basis for managing chronic diseases, including obesity, is medical nutrition therapy.[55,56] Medical nutrition therapy shouldn't, however, be used in isolation to treat obesity since compensatory brain mechanisms that increase appetite and ultimately lead to weight gain make it difficult to maintain weight loss over the long run.[57,58] Instead, medical nutrition therapy should be customized to fulfill a person's health- or weight-related goals in conjunction with other interventions (psychological, pharmacologic, or surgical).[56,59]

Typically, 3% to 5% of body weight can be lost with healthy behavioral adjustments, which can significantly reduce the comorbidities associated with obesity.[60] Individual differences in weight loss are significant and are influenced by biological, psychological, and other factors in addition to personal effort. The "best weight"—which may not correspond to an "ideal" weight on the BMI scale—is the weight at which the body maintains stability when participating in healthy behaviors. The "ideal" BMI may be quite challenging to attain. More intensive pharmacologic and surgical therapy alternatives can be taken into consideration if additional weight loss is required to improve health and well-being beyond what can be accomplished with behavioral adjustment.

behavioral and psychological therapies All health interventions, including methods for maintaining a healthy weight and level of physical activity, maintaining medication compliance, or preparing for and managing surgery, depend on changing behavior.61 Interventions in psychology and behavior are the "how to" of change. They give the clinician the ability to direct the patient toward suggested behaviors that are long-lasting.60 The chapter titled "Effective psychological and behavioral interventions in obesity management" may be found online (obesitycanada.ca/guidelines/) and provides a detailed discussion of psychological and behavioral interventions along with supporting data.

Pharmacotherapy For people with a BMI of 30 kg/m2 or a BMI of 27 kg/m2 with adiposity-related problems, we advise adjunctive medication for weight loss and weight-loss maintenance to enhance medical nutrition therapy, physical activity, and psychosocial interventions. Liraglutide 3.0 mg, orlistat, and a naltrexone-bupropion combo are available. Pharmacotherapy is crucial in preventing weight gain since it increases the magnitude of weight loss beyond what healthy behavior modifications alone can accomplish.62-66 The chapter titled "Pharmacotherapy in obesity management" may be found online (http://obesitycanada.ca/guidelines/) and provides a comprehensive description and supporting data.

Weight loss surgery For those with a BMI of 40 kg/m2 or below who also have at least one obesity-related illness, bariatric surgery may be an option. A multidisciplinary team should decide which type of surgery is best for the patient while weighing their expectations, the patient's health, and the potential advantages and disadvantages of the procedure. The chapters labeled "Bariatric Surgery: selection and preoperative workup," "Bariatric Surgery: options and outcomes," and "Bariatric surgery: postoperative management" are all available online at http://obesitycanada.ca/guidelines/ and provide a comprehensive description and supporting documentation.

Step 4: Agreeing on the therapy's objectives

Since obesity is a chronic illness, patient-provider cooperation is necessary for long-term management.67 Healthcare professionals should consult with their patients to establish reasonable expectations, person-centered care, and long-term objectives for behavior modification and health outcomes.68

Focusing on behavioral interventions to improve overall health, explicitly acknowledging the multiple factors that influence weight-disrupting stereotypes of personal failure or success attached to body composition, and redefining success as healthy behavior change regardless of body size or weight are all effective ways to reduce anti fat stigma in primary care consultations.69

Because this illness is chronic, a lengthy treatment regimen is required. A personalized action plan that tackles the causes of weight gain should be created by healthcare professionals and patients and agreed upon.70

Step 5: Advocacy and follow-up

Promoting more efficient care for those who are obese is necessary. Providing effective, scientifically supported care for obesity, entails enhancing the education and lifelong learning of healthcare professionals. To enhance access to efficient behavioral, pharmacologic, and surgical therapy alternatives, we must also support the allocation of health care resources. Significant obstacles are preventing Canadians from receiving adequate treatment for obesity. These obstacles include a severe lack of interdisciplinary programs for managing obesity, inadequate access to healthcare professionals with experience treating obese patients, lengthy wait times for referrals and surgery, and the high cost of some treatments.,37,71-73 Healthcare personnel are generally ill-equipped to handle obesity. 74 None of the existing anti-obesity drugs in Canada are covered by any provincial public drug benefit or pharmacare program, nor are any of them listed as a benefit on any provincial or territorial formulary.71 The longest wait periods for any surgically curable ailment are for bariatric surgery in Canada.37,71 Bariatric surgery is still not widely available in the majority of Canadian provinces and the three territories, despite some regions of the country seeing an increase in access to it. When a patient is referred for bariatric surgery, they may have to wait up to 8 years before seeing a specialist or having the procedure.

The rising rates of extreme obesity in Canada are a result of the lack of access to obesity therapies.46 Many weight-loss products and services lack a scientific basis and outright advocate for unattainable, unsustainable weight-loss objectives, leaving Canadians who are affected by obesity to traverse a confusing environment of weight-loss products and services.76

Methods

composition of the groups taking part

The executive committee and steering committee were put together by Obesity Canada and the Canadian Association of Bariatric Physicians and Surgeons with a wide range of expertise and geographic representation. The executive committee, which included two co-chairs (S.W. and D.C.W.L.), a primary care physician (D.C.-S.), a psychologist (M.V.), a bariatric surgeon (L.B.), and a nephrologist (A.M.S.), offered overall guidance and direction for the development of the guidelines.

The steering committee (n = 16) chose additional researchers (chapter heads and writers) to write each chapter. This group also included a person who struggles with obesity. In April 2017 and December 2017, the executive committee and steering committee met in person. They also spoke on the phone at least once a month.

Based on their experience in clinical practice and research in the field of obesity medicine, chapter leads and chapter authors (n = 60) were chosen for the chapters. There were between two and four authors per chapter. Chapter heads selected extra writers to contribute to each chapter's composition.

By having the Public Engagement Committee of Obesity Canada participate, we reached out to people who live with obesity (n = 7). The steering group for this guideline was given a Public Engagement group (I.P.) member (I.P.). Every month, the Public Engagement Committee held a phone meeting. Through focus groups, private chats, and online questionnaires, we collected contributions from committee members.

A focus group (n = 14) was used to recruit members of the indigenous community. Additionally, through a consensus-building process between these physicians and the chapter authors throughout the spring of 2019, we gained the perspectives of healthcare professionals working with Indigenous communities, which further anchored the data in clinical practice. Information can be found online at obesitycanada.ca/guidelines/ in the chapter titled "Obesity Management with Indigenous Peoples."

Staff members, consultants, and volunteers from Obesity Canada (n = 15) helped with project coordination and administrative support during the preparation of the guidelines. The duties of each group of participants are described in Table 2 along with the process used to generate the guidelines.

Table 2: Process for developing guidelines in summary

Activity Accountable group
• A mind-mapping activity to determine the broad divisions and chapters (19 chapters) and the guidelines' scopeExecutive board
• Create research questions for each chapter (PICO[T]).the steering group
• Research the literature 77 MERST
• Upload the Distiller Systematic Review software application MERST with the findings of the literature search.
• Evaluate every paper critically 77 section headings
• Examine the findings of the critical evaluation and, using the AGREE II tool, rate each paper based on the evidence.MERST • Create reports with graded evidence MERST • Create recommendations based on the

best available data and consensus among expertsSteering Committee includes writers and chapter leads

• Check suggestions to make sure they are consistent with the evidence (only for recommendations utilizing evidence of grades A–C).MERST • Examine recommendations to make sure they are consistent with the available data and pertinent to primary care medical practitioners. Executive Board

• Modify suggestions in light of input from the executive committee and MERST. Chapter leads on the steering committee

• Examine and accept the last recommendations. Executive Board

• External evaluation of proposals to determine their applicability and relevancePatients with obesity treated by family doctors and chapters that have undergone external peer review experts in every field

Note: PICO(T) is for Population, Intervention, Comparison, Outcome, and Time. AGREE stands for Appraisal of Guidelines for Research and Evaluation.

choice of high-priority subjects

To determine the scope of the guideline and the major sections and chapters (April–June 2017), the executive committee engaged in a mind-mapping exercise of 79 19 distinct sections and chapters were given priority. At a face-to-face meeting on December 15–16, 2017, the steering committee created PI/PECOT (Population, Intervention or Exposure, Comparison, Outcome, Time) questions for each chapter, yielding 179 questions to direct the literature search. The McMaster Evidence Review and Synthesis Team (MERST; formerly the McMaster Evidence-Based Practice Centre) provided support in developing all clinical questions in the proper format (e.g., PICO [T] for medicines and treatments, PEO for qualitative questions).

Review of the literature and quality evaluation

Through literature searches based on the PI/PECOT questions for each chapter, the McMaster

Evidence Review and Synthesis Team assisted in the formulation of the guidelines. Using this data, a health sciences librarian from Hamilton, Ontario's McMaster Health Sciences Library developed search algorithms for the MEDLINE and Embase databases. The searches covered peer-reviewed, released, and English-language literature from January 2006 to June 2018. In addition to the 7 searches that helped put the various chapters in context, 14 searches directly mapped to the chapters. On the obesity guidelines website (obesitycanada.ca/guidelines/), search techniques are accessible. The final collection of citations was sent to DistillerSR software for selection and review after the search results were uploaded to EndNote, where the duplicates had been deleted.80 The chapter authors also found additional citations and included them in the main search results in addition to the electronic searches.

Two reviewers independently chose research for inclusion after screening the publication titles and abstracts. Any citation that either reviewer decided to include was moved to the full-text review stage. One or more authors of the pertinent chapter examined full-text publications to determine their applicability. The Shekelle methodology was then used to evaluate the methodological quality of the chosen citations.[77,81] Each reference was divided into four categories: prognosis, evaluation of diagnostic qualities, and prevention. Following that decision, the relevant methods worksheet was displayed in the DistillerSR platform, where the methodological questions were resolved and an evidence level depending on the nature and caliber of the study was generated. The techniques worksheets (Box 3) were used to develop the levels of evidence, which were used to determine the strength of the recommendations.[77]

Box 3: Evidence categories77 Classification schemes

*Evidence derived from randomized controlled trials (RCTs) at Level 1a
*Evidence from at least one RCT at Level 1b
 *Level 2a: Support from at least one non randomized controlled research
*Evidence at Level 3 comes from non-experimental descriptive research including case-control, correlation, and comparison studies.
*Evidence at Level 4 includes reports from expert committees, expert committee judgments, respected authorities' clinical expertise, or both.

Strength of the advice

Directly based on level 1 evidence, grade A.
Grade B: Based solely on category 1 evidence or extrapolated from level 2 evidence.
Grade C: Based solely on level 3 evidence or extrapolated from

level 1 or 2 evidence with support.

Grade D: Directly based on evidence at level 4 or extrapolated suggestion from evidence at levels 1, 2, or 3.

This work has been modified with BMJ Publishing Group Limited's consent. Creating clinical guidelines. Shekelle PG, Woolf SH, Eccles M, et al. 1999;170:348–51; West J Med.

the creation of recommendations

The steering committee, chapter heads, and chapter authors developed recommendations based on the best available data (Box 3) The study reference that provided the highest level of support for the particular suggestion was added after the chapter leads and writers 77 examined the type and strength of the available evidence (level). Content experts in qualitative research (S.K., X.R.S., D.C.S., L.C., and S.R.M.) were involved in the examination of all the materials forming the basis of these recommendations because they recognize the value of qualitative research in addressing concerns relevant to the care of persons living with obesity. The level of evidence in these recommendations was based on a consensus assessment of the quality of the evidence by reviewers with knowledge of qualitative methodologies.

Some grade D suggestions were made based on expert committee findings, the views of renowned authorities, or clinical experience, and they were referenced as such. Other grade D recommendations were made by the writers of the chapter and were indicated with "Consensus" following the grade D.

To make the recommendation more specific, the chapter authors employed standardized vocabulary. The literature (Table 3) served as a basis for the actionable verbs utilized for each of the recommendations.82-84

Table 3: Actionable verb definitions utilized in the recommendations

Grade range recommended terms

Grade A recommendations at Level 1. Put the word "should" here.
Grade B recommendations at Level 2. Make use of the words "may" or "can"
Grade C recommendations at Level 3. Make use of the word "recommend"
4. Level 4, a D, and generally accepted suggestions"Suggest" should be used.
The recommendations were finalized through an iterative process. The clarity of the language and the integrity of the recommendations to the evidence were assessed for recommendations that received a grade between A and C by methodologists from MERST. Each recommendation was examined by two methodologists (primary and secondary reviewers), who used checklists

to determine the level of support for each citation. The methodologists got together, debated, and came to an agreement on how to grade the recommendations. They then gave their proposals to the executive committee for changes to the language or grading. Based on the MERST review procedure, the chapter amended the recommendations.

To ensure agreement, the executive committee cast votes on each recommendation. If there was not unanimous support for a recommendation, the executive committee debated it extensively until there was. The chapter leads later changed this recommendation's phrasing as necessary, and the executive committee approved the revised version. All of the recommendations received final approval from the executive committee. This guideline's recommendations all received unanimous support.

External evaluation

The recommendations were evaluated for relevance and viability by outside reviewers (primary care physicians and obese individuals [n = 7]). To represent the language and the primary care setting, we made certain changes. For every chapter, a separate external peer review was done.

control of conflicting interests
The Canadian Association of Bariatric Physicians and Surgeons, the Canadian Institutes of Health Research Strategic Patient-Oriented Research initiative, Obesity Canada's Fund for Obesity Collaboration and Unified Strategies (FOCUS) initiative, and in-kind contributions from the scientific and professional volunteers involved in the process provided the funding. The guidelines' content has not been impacted by the funding organization's opinions. Chapter leads, chapter authors and members of the executive and steering committees were all volunteers who received no payment for their work.

The competing interest policy and procedures for reducing bias were created and handled by the executive committee. On the

website for the guidelines, you
can find the policy and
disclosures of competing
interests. Everyone who took part
had to declare any potential
conflicting interests. We
continuously updated the steering
and executive committee
members' statements of potential
conflicts of interest, as well as
those of the participating
MERST methodologists. We
included information about
government funding sources in
the disclosure form created by
the International Committee of
Medical Journal Editors.
No one with relevant disclosures
was barred from participating in
the critical evaluations or voting
on the recommendations.
However, the executive
committee requested that those
who had direct conflicts of
interest abstain from voting in
certain areas. Any mention of the
off-label usage of medications
always carried the disclaimer that
it was off-label.
To make sure the evidence had
been fairly evaluated,
methodologists from MERST
who had no conflicting interests

reviewed and graded each
included study. To make sure
that the suggestions were in line
with the evidence, they also
assessed the recommendations
(rated between A and C). To
determine whether the proposals
were feasible and to check for
bias, we ultimately performed an
external review procedure.

Implementation

The Canadian Association of
Bariatric Surgeons and
Physicians and Obesity Canada
have collaborated to create a
website
(obesitycanada.ca/guidelines)
where the full guideline, interim
updates, a quick reference guide,
key messages, resources for
health care providers, slide kits,
videos, and webinars, as well as
information for those who are
obese and the people who
support them, are all available in
both English and French. The
policy will be kept up to date and
hosted on the website. Each
chapter lead will keep track of
the evidence supporting this
proposal, and they will work
with the executive committee to
update the recommendations

whenever new information becomes available that might change them. Appendix 2 contains a framework for implementation known as the 5As Framework.

Access to obesity care is still a problem in Canada more than ten years after the first Canadian obesity guidelines were published in 2006. Despite statements from the Canadian Medical Association85 and the World Health Organization, the federal, provincial, territorial, and municipal governments do not formally acknowledge obesity as a chronic condition.86 Access to treatment is hampered by the failure of public and commercial payers, healthcare systems, the general public, and the media to recognize obesity as a chronic condition.72 The fact that obesity is still viewed as a self-inflicted disease has an impact on the interventions and strategies that are used by governments or are funded by health benefit programs.87 The implementation of this recommendation will call for focused policy action, advocacy work, and involvement from individuals with obesity, their families, and healthcare professionals. Organizations in Canada have banded together to alter the perception of obesity in the country, to end stigma associated with obesity and weight bias, and to alter the way healthcare institutions and policies treat obesity.88 This recommendation will be used to support lobbying efforts on behalf of the federal and provincial governments to enhance the treatment of obese people.

The following rules
The first Canadian clinical practice guideline based on evidence for the prevention and treatment of obesity in adults and children was published in 2006.43 A set of recommendations for the prevention of weight gain and the use of behavioral and pharmaceutical interventions to manage overweight and obesity in adults in primary care were released in 2015 by the Canadian Task Force on Preventive Health Care in collaboration with the

scientific staff of the Public Health Agency of Canada and the McMaster Evidence Review and Synthesis Centre.89 This guideline only examined intervention trials carried out in settings generalizable to Canadian primary care, and it was not intended to "apply to people with BMI of 40 or greater, who may benefit from specialized bariatric programs." Also excluded from the recommendation were surgical procedures.

gaps in understanding

The best level of evidence that was available in 2020 served as the basis for the recommendations in this guideline. We acknowledge that continued research will help to improve and inform the management of obesity.90,91 Except for surgical intervention, current treatment approaches seldom result in sustained weight loss of more than 20%, and for some persons who are obese, this amount of weight loss may not be sufficient to resolve or alleviate many adiposity-related medical issues. To satisfy the requirements of those who are obese, more treatment alternatives are required. For many people who have received treatment, weight regain remains a challenge.92

Conclusion

In Canada and around the world, obesity is a common, complicated chronic disease that affects many individuals. However, only a small percentage of those who need treatment for their obesity have access to it. This revised evidence-based recommendation aims to improve access and care for persons who are obese by encouraging medical professionals to acknowledge the need for long-term treatment. The more recent understanding of how appetite is regulated and the pathophysiology of obesity have opened up new treatment options for this chronic illness. Raising the bar for care and enhancing the well-being of those who live with obesity will require reducing weight bias and stigma, comprehending the underlying causes of obesity, and encouraging and supporting patient-centered behavioral interventions and appropriate treatment by healthcare professionals, preferably with the assistance of interdisciplinary care teams. Our objectives to combat this common chronic condition include the dissemination and application of this guideline. To close the information gaps, much more work needs to be put into research, education, prevention, and treatment of obesity.

Acknowledgments

The construction of the Obesity Guidelines website, online tools, tables, and figures was made possible by the coordination support provided by Obesity Canada employees Dawn Hatanaka, Nicole Pearce, Brad Hussey, Robert Fullerton, and Patti Whitefoot-Bobier. The authors also acknowledge Lisa Schaffer, Candace Vilhan, Kelly Moen, Doug Earle, and

Brenndon Goodman of the Obesity Canada Public Engagement Committee, who reviewed key messages for people with obesity and suggestions for healthcare professionals and helped to develop the research questions. The authors also acknowledge Donna Fitzpatrick, a member of the McMaster Evidence Review and Synthesis Team (MERST), who was essential in creating the techniques required for the guideline, as well as the reviewers whose suggestions contributed to enhancing the chapters and this publication. Elham Kamran and Rubin Pooni provided research help, while Jordan Tate from the Physician Learning Program at the University of Alberta created the 5As framework for the guideline. The authors also thank Brad Hussey and Barbara Kermode-Scott for revising the recommendations.